YOUR KNOWLEDGE HAS VALUE

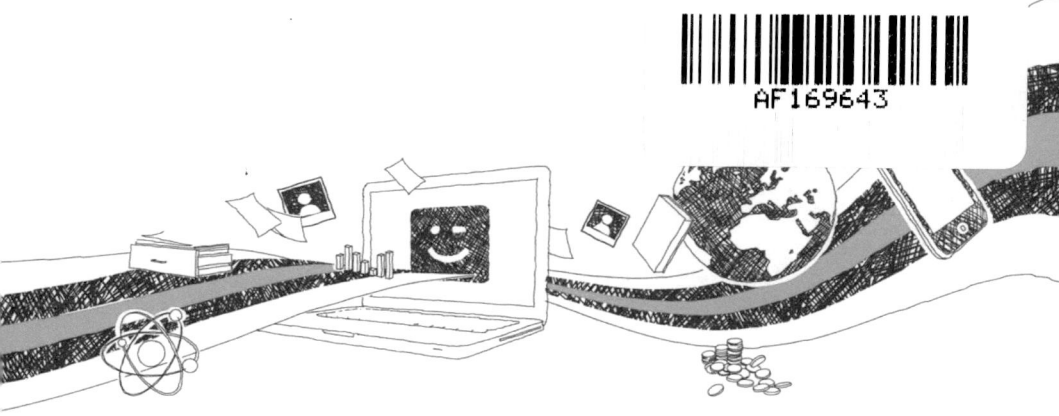

- We will publish your bachelor's and master's thesis, essays and papers

- Your own eBook and book - sold worldwide in all relevant shops

- Earn money with each sale

Upload your text at www.GRIN.com
and publish for free

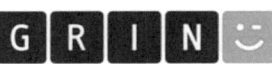

Bibliographic information published by the German National Library:

The German National Library lists this publication in the National Bibliography; detailed bibliographic data are available on the Internet at http://dnb.dnb.de .

This book is copyright material and must not be copied, reproduced, transferred, distributed, leased, licensed or publicly performed or used in any way except as specifically permitted in writing by the publishers, as allowed under the terms and conditions under which it was purchased or as strictly permitted by applicable copyright law. Any unauthorized distribution or use of this text may be a direct infringement of the author s and publisher s rights and those responsible may be liable in law accordingly.

Imprint:

Copyright © 2015 GRIN Verlag, Open Publishing GmbH
Print and binding: Books on Demand GmbH, Norderstedt Germany
ISBN: 9783668456594

This book at GRIN:

http://www.grin.com/en/e-book/366971/menstrual-hygiene-management-in-refugee-camps-a-qualitative-assessment

Wudalew Meselu Tesfaye

Menstrual Hygiene Management in Refugee Camps. A Qualitative Assessment using Focus Group Discussions

GRIN Publishing

GRIN - Your knowledge has value

Since its foundation in 1998, GRIN has specialized in publishing academic texts by students, college teachers and other academics as e-book and printed book. The website www.grin.com is an ideal platform for presenting term papers, final papers, scientific essays, dissertations and specialist books.

Visit us on the internet:

http://www.grin.com/

http://www.facebook.com/grincom

http://www.twitter.com/grin_com

Management of Menstrual Hygiene among Women living in Bokolmanyo Refugee Camp

25th Dec, 2013

alew Meseln

Contents

Introduction 3
Objective of the FGD 3
Methodology 4
Key Findings of the FGD 5
Results of the FGD 6
Conclusion and recommendations 11
Annex I 12
A Guideline for Focus Group Discussion on Menstrual Hygiene Management (MHM) for women living in Bokolmanyo Camp 12

Annex.II-Questionnaire 13

Introduction

Many literatures had mentioned that **MENSTRUAL HYGIENE** has been largely neglected by WASH sectors and others focusing on sexual and reproductive health, and education. As a result millions of women and girly continue to be denied of their rights for WASH, health, education, dignity and gender equity. Though it is a natural part of the reproductive cycle, menstruation, in most parts of the world, it remains a taboo and is rarely talked about. Thus, the practical challenges of menstrual hygiene are made even more difficult by various socio cultural factors.

The provision of sanitary materials is crucial not only to the health of women and girls, but also to their dignity and protection. While the High Commissioner's five commitments to Refugee Women includes the provision of sanitary materials to all women and girls of concern, the available data shows that this commitment has been fulfilled only in one third of the operations worldwide. (UNHCR Guidelines to Hygiene Promotion, March 2011)

Lack of involvement in decision making, lack of information and awareness, poor or no access to products and facilities, and lack of social support were found as the major factors for the poor menstrual hygiene.

Recognizing that, the factors affecting menstrual hygiene of women are different in different settings/contexts, the investigator conducted two Focus Group Discussions (24 discussants); with Child bearing women in the camp and girls (15-18 years) who are attending schools with the aim to identify the access to MHM materials, challenges and the utilization behaviors of the refugees and assess their preference to the type of MHM materials.

Objective of the FGD
- To assess women's previous/before coming to the camps/ experiences regarding menstrual hygiene management
- To assess women's practice of MHM items
- To identify women's preference towards the types of sanitary pads
- To identify the challenges women are facing in addressing MH needs
- To understand the awareness of school girls regarding menstrual hygiene

alew Meselu

Methodology

Study Period
- This focus group discussion was conducted 13th December 2013 – 14th December 2013.

Study area
- These focus group discussions were conducted at Bokolmanyo refugee camp.

Study population/Discussants
- The participants of the focus group discussion were women of child bearing age residing in Bokolmanyo refugee camp and Females (age greater than 15) attending school.

Two FGDs comprising of women of child bearing age and female school attendants with a total number of 24 discussants were conducted.

Table 1 FGD discussants

Name of the FGD	Discussion participants	Number of discussants
FGD 1	Women association members and Refugee Community Members	12
FGD 2	Female Students of child bearing age	12

Participants of the FGDs were selected with consent. Appointments were made with the selected volunteers/discussants as where and when the discussion was going to be held. Then the discussion was held as per the pre-determined time and place

Key Findings of the FGD

- Different experiences of sanitary pads utilization were observed among the discussants before their arrival to the camp. Those women coming from urban area used had the experience of sanitary pads utilization while those women coming from rural part of Somalia used to use clothes.

- Reusable Clothes and sanitary pads were used as the main menstrual hygiene materials as most of the discussants explained. One of the discussants says "...before my arrival to this camp, I used to use cloths and currently I use sanitary pads to manage my periodic menstruation".

- Almost all of the discussants were found to be expertise in using the sanitary pads. Many discussants stated that they currently use clothes pointing that sanitary pads could not easily be accessed by them.

- "We know that MHM materials are essential for us but we currently are not accessing them, we have received them long time ago and thus we are in a problem to manage our periodic menstruation" said a woman among the discussants indicting that there is a great demand for MHM items by the refugees.

- The Disposable type sanitary pad was preferred by majority of the discussants putting their fear of the health costs that the reusable type sanitary pad would boast on them.

alew Meselu

Results of the FGD
Feelings of women upon arrival to the camps

Most of the discussants were quite responsive when answering "What things did you feel you need for you hygiene and health upon your arrival to the camp?" Very few of them keep quite from responding to the question. Most of the discussant's thought that drugs were the first priorities for their health while water, water collection jerry cans, latrines, and soap were priority demands for hygiene. Limited number of discussants mentioned; basins, potties and sanitary pads as essential items for their personal hygiene. One of the discussants said. "When I first arrived in this camp, the first thing that I felt as essential for me and my family was medicine, water and jerry cans and soap for health and hygiene."

Hygiene and health information were seldom given to most of the respondents. *"Upon my arrival to the camp, there was no body coming me to provide health and hygiene messages."* Some of them also mentioned that *"...this is the first time to sit in a circle and discuss on menstrual hygiene".*

On the other hand, few discussants said that health and hygiene messages were delivered to them upon their arrival to the camp. *"Discussions regarding environmental hygiene/cleanness and the utilization of sanitary pads were conducted by ARRA Corps."*

Women's menstrual hygiene practice before coming to the camps

It was observed that the existing cultural differences between the rural and the urban population in Somalia have contributed to the MHM practices of women. Discussants stated that, most of the women coming from urban area used sanitary pads while those originating from rural part of Somalia used to use clothes to manage their periodic menstruation. *"I myself came from urban area, thus I have been using sanitary pads."* On the other hand, a woman from rural area replied that she used to use cloth for managing her MH.

Access to MHM items and Current Utilization/practice of women

Women and girls often find menstrual hygiene difficult due to a lack of access to appropriate sanitary protection products or facilities. Currently, in Bokolmanyo camp most of the respondents have been found using cloths for menstrual hygiene. This was because of the lack of sanitary pads. Lack of access to sanitary pads was cited as a problem by all of the discussants and thus they are using clothes instead of sanitary pads during their menstruation.

Discussants were asked about the access to MHM items. Almost all of the respondents reported that they used to access the MHM items previously from ARRA together with the ration they were receiving monthly. The distribution of these items had been made by ARRA long time ago. *"MHM items were consecutively distributed for about 4 times in the last years, though we have received them long time ago."*

Discussants explained that MHM materials are essential for them and they showed a great demand for. It was understood from the FGD that women are in challenge of their MH due to the lack of MHM items and the in affordability of the items by women. "MHM items are like our daily intake, we cannot afford the cost for them and thus a challenge to manage our periodic menstruation."

Participants of the FGD were also asked to explain the way how they received the MHM items. They briefed like this, "...there were workers coming to our zone/home to take our list. Then after completing the list of the beneficiaries, distribution was made according to our family size i.e priority was given for those families with larger sizes and then to the smaller size families"

Most of the women/discussants reported that they were not able to buy the items by themselves while very few of them said that they were able to purchase the items from the market whenever available.

All of the discussants mentioned that they know how to use the items, though their accessibility is the challenge women are currently facing in the camp.

MHM items Utilization behavior of women

Currently, reusable Cloth was usually used by most of the discussants. "We were using reusable cloth. By the time we want to change the cloth once used, change it with a clean one and wash the one used for the next day/time."

The difference between sanitary pads and the cloth was not perceived as significant by some of the discussants. They justify that the reusable cloth is preferable because it can easily be accessed while the sanitary pads could not be accessed.

alew Meselu

Women were also asked to explain how the displacement affected their MHM needs. Most of them quite answered the question. They talked about the challenges they faced during their journey to Ethiopia. Since they didn't carry the item during the displacement, women were in a problem during their journey to the camps; "...my cloth was stained by my blood and I was embarrassed since I was walking together with men. The pain was also the very bad condition I was challenged off during the displacement/emergency" says one the women among discussants.

Appropriateness of the MHM items for women

MHM Items were perceived by most of the respondents as essential items to manage their menstruation. The availability of these items was a great concern for the discussion participants. Though some items like, water and soap for cleaning were available; the essential ones i.e sanitary pads and pants were missing items as most of the discussion participants mentioned.

Discussants were asked what things to be improved for the future to better manage their menstruation. They said that the priority action should be making the items avail for us, "currently were have no sanitary pads to use, thus we are in great demand of them."

Type of MHM items and women's preference

Both types of the sanitary pads (disposable and reusable) were presented for the discussants. Astonishingly, all of the discussants' preference was for the disposable type of the sanitary pad. They were asked to justify why they choose the disposable one. They mentioned their fear of the infections (RTI and UTIs) and other health consequences they may suffer from using the reusable sanitary pad.

Women's safety during MHM Items Distribution

This FGD showed that women were not feeling safe during distribution of MHM Items. Three reasons were mentioned for this;

- Due to a large crowd of people coming for the distribution, there will be long waiting time to receive the items
- Priorities were not given for the vulnerable people like; pregnant women, lactating mothers, women with disabilities.
- No shelter for distribution.

For the above mentioned problems that were observed during distribution, the following recommendations were forwarded by the discussants as corrective measures for their safety @ distribution.

alew Meselu

- *Giving priority for the vulnerable women/ladies*
- *Distributing the items together with hygiene kits so that it can reduce the shame women are feeling*

Facilities and disposal options used by women for MHM

Latrines were used as facilities/places where most of the women ware changing/replacing the used sanitary pads. The discussants were also asked if they have a space for washing and drying of used towels/reusable sanitary pads. Their response was, 'No'. Proper management of the used sanitary pads or under wears is the responsibility of WASH implementing partners. Unsafe disposal of sanitary pads could have a risk of infecting other people if they come in contact with; especially Hepatitis B. For that reason, women need to have facilities for safely disposing used sanitary pads or a place to dry them if they are reusable.

The disposal practice in Bokolmanyo is that almost all of discussants responses were similar saying that they are disposing the used sanitary pads in the latrines. *"...I drop it in to the latrine; because it is waste."* Some others considered the used sanitary pads as feces and drop it in the latrine. Few of them reported that they were burying it in a small pit. Among those who used to dispose in a latrine, some of them explained their interest in burying in a small pit understanding the drawbacks of disposing in a latrine.

Water availability for MHM and protection issues were also raised during the discussion. It is recommended that sex segregated latrines are required to promote proper disposal of the used sanitary pads. Though, this was not the case in Bokolmanyo camp, the women have the adopted using those available latrines. The challenge mentioned by some of the discussants was lack of light in the latrines to make women feel safety during the night time.

The following recommendations were forwarded by the discussants as actions to improve MHM for the future;
- To have sex segregated latrines with water connection
- Uninterrupted availability of the items
- Provision of soap including other hygiene kits like towel, shampoo and tooth brush with paste

alew Meselu

Awareness of school girls regarding menstrual hygiene

Young girls often grow up with limited knowledge of menstruation because their mothers and other women shy away from discussing the issues within them. Not only for the girls but also it is important for men to understand the menstrual hygiene so they can support their wives, mothers, daughters, and students.

This FGD showed that students had good awareness of menstrual hygiene and the natural process. *"When a girl's body becomes large and starts menstruating, then she is becoming a matured adult/woman."* said one of the girls. Most of the girls were aware that they defined menstruation period as a **monthly cycle of blood flow** when a girls gets matured.

MHM items utilization behavior of School girls

Most of the girls reported they have the experience of using sanitary pads. The use of clothes to manage menstrual blood flow was also practiced by few of the girls. As mentioned by most of the discussants, sanitary pads were preferred than the cloth as the sanitary pad is more comfortable. *"I feel more comfortable when I use a sanitary pad than cloth"*

The very interesting thing was that school attendance by these students was not influence by menstruation. Students reported *"we attend school during our menstruation period"*.

The latrines built for students are sex segregated which makes it safer for them to manage their menstrual hygiene. *Though sex segregated, latrines were not connected with water that could be a challenge for girls when they need to clean themselves and change sanitary pads.*

Information demand of School girls

- **Counseling sessions in the school and**
- **Provision of awareness to mothers;** were mentioned as better ways to address the demands of school girls for menstrual hygiene information.

Conclusion and recommendations

- It was identified that may of the discussants had few exposures to discuss menstrual hygiene issues. Thus, group discussions by female CHPs/CHWs and other means of information provision need to be considered to improve better utilization and disposal of the sanitary pads.
- As the Higher Commissioner's FIVE Commitments to refugee Women includes the provision of sanitary materials to all women and girls of concern. It will be good if the WASH sector and other partners give more attention (besides UNHCR's Concern) to address the women's demand for MHM items. The disposable type of the sanitary pads was the preferred MHM item.
- For the better safety of women and the vulnerable, it is recommendable to construct a shelter for the distribution of MHM items
- In addition to the MHM items, constant provision of soap and other personal hygiene items will improve the proper management of menstrual hygiene
- Most of the women showed their demand for sex segregated latrines with water connection and lights around the latrines to keep their safety
- Distribution of items shall be done together with the other hygiene kits so that the shame among women will be reduced.
- It is recommendable to connect school's latrines with water for the better management of girls' menstrual hygiene.
- Counseling sessions for students and provision of awareness to mothers will be important to improve menstrual hygiene management among school girls

alew Meselu

Annex I

A Guideline for Focus Group Discussion on Menstrual Hygiene Management (MHM) for women living in Bokolmanyo Camp

Hello, my name is …. We are conducting focus group discussions on Menstrual Hygiene Management (MHM). The results of this discussion will be used to develop appropriate and feasible strategies for the better utilization and disposal of MHM items in this camp. The discussion will take about an hour.

Participation in this survey is voluntary and you have unreserved right not to discuss issues you thought not relevant and important. If you don't understand any of the discussion points, please feel free to ask for clarification. I really think a lot for your willingness and time to be with us for this discussion. Shall we start the discussion and record it with tape now? If ok proceed.

Annex II

Questionnaire for FGD on Menstrual Hygiene Management for women living in Bokolmanyo Camp

1. Think about when you first arrived in (here/camp/location). What things did you feel you and your family needed for your health or hygiene requirements?

2. Were you able to get these items (or support)?

   PROBE: How did you obtain the items and/or support? Have ever bought these items by your own? How often? Where did you buy them? Were facilities (water, latrines etc) available?

3. At any point after you arrived, did anybody ever ask you about the health and hygiene of you or your family, or what you needed to improve your health? For example, did anyone ever bring you into a circle like this to ask you what you needed?

   PROBE: If yes, who asked you? What did they ask? Who else did they ask? Was the support you asked provided?

4. Before coming to the camp, what do you normally use to manage your menstrual cycle? (Highlight if support other than personal sanitary items are brought out but don't bring it out …. It will be drawn out later)

   PROBE: Ask participants to describe items they used? What material – clothes, locally produced sanitary pads…?

5. After arriving in the camp, what are you using now to manage your menstrual cycle?

   PPROBE: what material are they using - reusable clothes, disposable pads . . .,
   If different from what they were using before to the camp, how that affected them? If same, is it easy to get the items now? How does the emergency/displacement affect your MHM needs? How did it feel not having these items/facilities?

6. Were you able to get personal MHM items?

   PROBE: how did you obtain the items? Who made the distribution? How often? Were you able to buy these items by your own at times of absence of distribution? Did you or your family have to sacrifice buying other items? If not how do you manage your MHM needs? Were the items the same as what you regularly use? Were the items appropriate?

Probe: If so what were the differences? Why are there differences? Do they know how to use?

7. **Were the MHM items appropriate,**

    PROBE: do facilities are available for better MHM? What facilities are missing? What do you want to see changed for better MHM?

8. **Which type of MHM items you think is appropriate? Why?** *Reusable Vs disposable-* . (in the group, get the number of those using reusable, disposable pads, both , others or nothing to get an indication of % usage)
    PROBE: is the choice based on absence of facilities, say if they choice disposable than reusable, ask them provision of which key facilities could change the choice or the choice based on economy/ cost... are there any health related reasons (are they aware of RTI or UTI) ...

9. **Tell me about the process of receiving menstrual hygiene items** */pads or clothes as applicable/*

    PROBE: who was doing the distribution? How did you hear about them? Did you or anyone else in the HH pick them up? Was this a problem? Why? How far is the distribution point from where you live? What problem that will have?

10. **Did you feel safe during the distribution?**

    PROBE: Why, Why not?

11. **How should women's hygiene items be distributed in the future?**

    PROBE: Should they be distributed with the kits, separately, through a facility? Why?

12. **Did you have the proper facilities for MHM?**

    PROBE: Where do you change your sanitary pads?
    Reusable/towels: *do you have space for washing and drying of towels? Do you thoroughly wash the cloth with soap? Do you dry it in the sun? How long do you use the same cloth? Where do you dispose the cloth?-. Is it appropriate?*
    Disposable pads: *where do you dispose of your pads? Do you see pads littered?*
    Water availability: *availability of separate/private functional latrines and water?*
    Protection: *are toilets lockable from the inside? Do you feel safe to use the latrines during the night?*

13. **Looking at your current situation, what type of changes or improvement to facilities are needed for your MHM?**

    PROBE: discuss what has been previously raised, discuss facilities requirement in priority

14. **After discussing all aspects of MHM where is the priority of support needed?**

alew Meselu

PROBE: Supply of Hygiene items, improvement to facilities ...

15. Is there anything else you would like to share about MHM?

With school girls:

1. What they know of becoming a woman? What does it mean?

    PROBE: Ask them what they know of menstrual cycle and who told them about it mother, grandmother, elders sister, auntie, teachers
2. What type of MHM items do you use? Why? (*Show samples if you can*) and which one do you prefer and why? Also try to get the % usage. (This can also be later compared with figures of older ladies above) what is the disposal methods
3. Do you come to school when you are menstruating? If not, why not?
4. What would make it easier to come to school when you are menstruating?
5. Are the toilet facilities at your school appropriate to deal with your menstrual flow? If you could change one thing about the toilets what would it be?
6. What kind of information would be useful for younger girls about to start menstruating?

YOUR KNOWLEDGE HAS VALUE

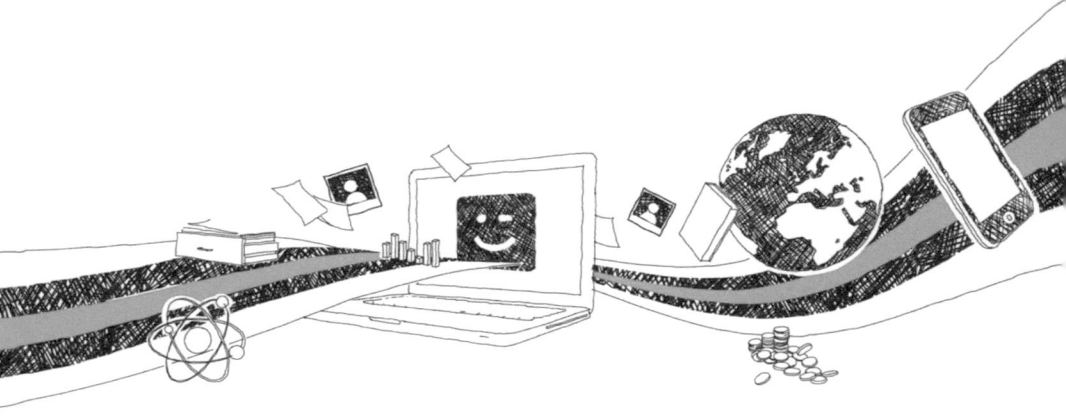

- We will publish your bachelor's and master's thesis, essays and papers

- Your own eBook and book - sold worldwide in all relevant shops

- Earn money with each sale

Upload your text at www.GRIN.com
and publish for free

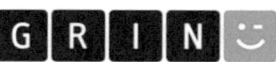